Natural Remedies For Beginners

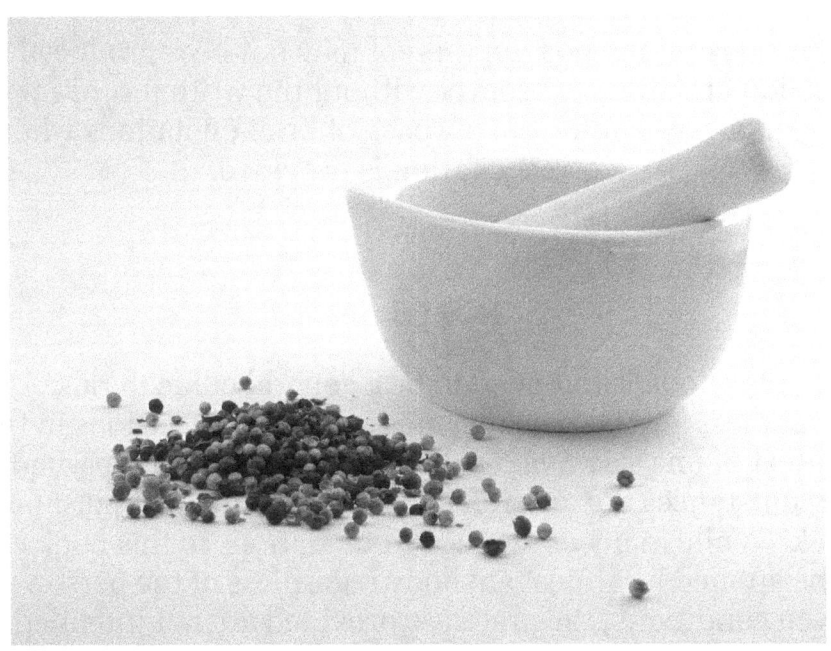

How To Protect, Cure And Beautify Yourself Without Prescriptions

By Dr Alex Nelson

Disclaimer

This book is intended to be a general guide to raise awareness and help people make informed decisions in the context of one's own personal circumstance. As everybody's circumstances are different, so are the remedies you should seek. While many of the recommendations in this book can be applied by almost anybody regardless of the person's given conditions, the practices provided are not intended to and should not be relied upon to replace professional medical advice.

The author accepts no responsibility for any loss or injury, be it personal or financial, as a result of the use or misuse of the information in this book. If you have any doubts or concerns, either while or after reading this book, please speak to a doctor or any other qualified person before taking any actions.

Contents

Introduction

Every species that inhabits the planet Earth can be considered very lucky. For starters, we have been given the opportunity to exist in a planet that is actually habitable, unlike other planets which are either too cold or too hot for living creatures to survive. We have also been endowed with a very rich environment, which is filled with natural resources and provisions from which both plants and animals could benefit. In short, the solution to all of our problems can be found in the very environment that we inhabit and everything that we could ever ask for has already been given to us by nature. Everything, in this context, consists of but is not limited to food, water, clothes, shelter, , protection, wealth, occupations, fun and recreation, love, and even cures to the diseases and illnesses which we acquire from time to time.

Speaking of natural cures and remedies, it is still a great mystery as to why a lot of people are still not open to the idea of using cures that come from plants and herbs, and instead prefer synthetically produced drugs over these natural cures. Apart from the fact that these synthetic drugs are expensive, they can also introduce toxins to our bodies. However, we still patronize these drugs and continually utilize them. We have already become a society that's dependent on synthetic drugs and is blind to the side-effects of these drugs.

One probable explanation for our neglect of natural cures is ignorance. We lack the necessary information about the benefits of using natural remedies and what the cures are,which is why we don't have faith in them. We often doubt the effectiveness and legitimacy of these remedies because we are accustomed to using synthetic drugs that are produced by multinational pharmaceuticals.

This ebook aims to open a new door for you, a door towards the appreciation of the natural remedies that even our ancestors have used since the beginning of history. This ebook also showcases the different natural cures and remedies that can aid the common ailments and diseases that we acquire in order to educate you about the healing powers of nature. The majority of these cures are highly accessible and can be easily purchased in the market or can even be found in your gardens. Some are just simple tips and procedures that you can easily follow to prevent acquiring some common diseases.

The main topic that will be talked about in Chapter 1 is the natural remedies that can cure mild infections like cough, cold, and sore throat.

Chapter 2, on the other hand, will tackle a more sophisticated set of conditions. It will talk about the natural cures to mental and neurological conditions like anxiety, depression, vertigo, and insomnia.

The natural remedy for gastrointestinal conditions is the main concept addressed in Chapter 3.

Chapter 4 will look into the ailments that affect the skin and other external conditions.

Chapter 5 will tell you how to battle daily ailments, the natural way.

And lastly, chapter 6 will give you skin care and health tips that you can follow in order to better take care of your children's health and well-being.

Chapter 1

Natural Remedies For Mild Infections

Among the most common infections that humans acquire every year include colds, cough, flu, and sore throat. These are the most prevalent reasons why people take an absence from jobs or school and are the main illnesses that employees use to explain why they are calling in sick from their responsibilities at work. The worst thing about these infections is that they don't choose the target. Anyone who has a weak immune system can be hit, no matter how young or old, or how poor or wealthy these people are.

Although these are just mild infections and are, almost often, not life threatening, they still cause us to feel tired and down. When these infections hit us, our bodies find it hard to function properly and perform our daily routines, and these can be great sources of annoyance and burden to most of us.

Now, you might be wondering: What causes these infections? How can they be cured or if not, prevented? What can we do to minimize the discomfort caused by these infections? This chapter will address all of those questions and teach you how to remedy these infections with the help of Mother Nature.

Common Cold

Colds are one of the leading illnesses that people acquire in every passing year. It is a common infection for the reason that there are a lot of viruses (almost 200 different strands and kinds of virus) that cause this ailment. The most popular virus that can cause colds is the rhinovirus and it accounts for at least 10 to 40 percent of the total number of cases of colds.

Getting a cold may not seem serious but it can cause you a great deal of discomfort and inconvenience, especially if you have important things to attend such as a major exam or a presentation of a big business proposal. It is not easy to think and do your chores properly if you have to constantly pause for a moment in order to sneeze or blow your nose.

Start and symptoms of a cold

Having a cold begins at the moment when you acquire the virus and your immune system fails to get rid of it. Once the virus overcomes the power of your immune systems, the cold virus then attaches itself to the linings of your nose or throat. It then confuses your cells to produce copies of the virus, thus causing them to multiply.

Usually, the symptoms to watch out for in order to determine that you are a victim of the cold virus are repeated and abnormal sneezing, an itchy or drippy nose, sore throat, congestion in the nasal area, watery and teary eyes, and or a fever and even muscles aches.

How can someone catch a cold?

So what can expose you to the possibility of catching a cold? There are multiple of causes for people to catch this virus. Firstly, the cold is the kind of infection that is highly contagious and spreads easily – that means being around someone or interacting with someone who has the cold virus can also make you vulnerable to the infection. The virus can be passed on through shaking a person's hand, kissing them, talking to them, or even just being around them when they unfortunately happened to sneeze. In other words, the cold virus can be passed on through body fluids.

There are also other precursors that can let you catch a cold. Some of these are fatigue and stress. Being constantly exposed to stressful environments or to people

4

who constantly make you stressed and tired can eventually lead to a weakened immune system. Stress can cause your built-in defences to crumble and when this happens, you cannot protect yourself from harmful bacteria and virus. These microorganisms can easily invade your body and cause havoc in your bodily systems.

The weather condition can also cause someone to have a cold. These days, the weather is somewhat moody. One moment it's sunny and then after a few hours, it suddenly rains. You just cannot predict the weather and when you are not ready for the instant change, you become prone to infections such as colds.

Another reason for which people catch colds is when they become exposed to things that trigger allergies. Once your allergies start to act up, colds usually follow.

Remedies

Most colds only last for 10 days. However, we do not want to suffer that long, do we? Here are some of the natural procedures that you can try in order to relieve the inconvenience that the cold virus can bring:

- *Rest*
  - When colds hit you, the best thing that you can do is rest. Yes. That means you have to take a little break from your work or from school. Further stressing and working up yourself will not do your immune system any good. You need to recharge your energy and allow your body to heal itself in order to battle the infection. Also, you will not be the only one who can benefit from your absence. You will also avoid passing the virus to others by staying in your bed and resting. Just imagine the discomfort if you really yourself force to take that Statistics test with a drippy nose or if you are

sneezing every five seconds in front of your boss. So, stay warm and comfortable in your bed to give yourself the chance to get better.

- ***Drink lots and lots of water***
  - The rule of thumb in treating a cold is to always rehydrate. When you sneeze and blow through your nose, you also lose body fluids and water. If you don't drink a lot of water, your throat and nose will become more irritated. Don't allow that to happen.

  - Drinking lots of water can also cause the mucus to become easier to flush out from your body, thus making it easier for your body to get rid of the virus.

- ***Steam it up***
  - When you have nasal congestion whenever you have a cold, it really is very hard to breathe. You can remedy this by inhaling some steam. The steam can ease the passage of air through your nostrils and passageways, helping you breathe more easily.

  - Like drinking lots of water, inhaling some steam can also help the mucus or the phlegm become softer and easier to blow out of your nose.

- ***Let it go***
  - One of the basic ways on how to get rid of your cold is to blow it out from your body. Don't keep it in your body, as it is not meant to be there. If you do keep it from coming out, the virus will spread and multiply in your body. However, it is

also imperative that you know how to blow your nose properly. Aggressive blowing can hurt your nose and it can get scratched in the process. When blowing your nose, you have to use soft tissue. Always avoid the rough ones. Also, make sure that you blow your nose gently so you don't strain the linings of your nose.

Food to eat

When you have a cold, you must make sure that you overload yourself with fruits that are rich in Vitamin C. You need Vitamin C in order to help your immune system fight the virus that causes the infection. So, it would be helpful if you munch on fruits like lemons and oranges. Hot soup can also help, especially if you have nasal congestion.   Please avoid cold water.

Omega-3 fatty acids have the power to lessen inflammations. So, if you have a cold, you can eat fish rich in omega-3 fatty acids like tuna. Also, you can eat some oysters because they contain zinc which battles against viruses that cause colds.

Cough

Coughing is a natural reflex that all of us do whenever there is something that irritates our throat. It is our body's way of eliminating foreign substances that cause irritation. However, coughing is not normal anymore when phlegm is already involved. The presence of phlegm when you cough already means that you are infected with a virus or bacteria.

There are generally two kinds of cough: acute and chronic cough. Acute cough only lasts for more or less 3 weeks while chronic cough can go for eight weeks or more.

Causes

Cough can be caused by a lot of factors. Like the cold, it is commonly caused by a respiratory tract infection brought about by a virus. However, a virus does not cause some cases of coughing, like in pneumonia. Instead, the culprits can be bacteria. Sometimes, cold, cough, and flu occur together and can make someone's life miserable.

The virus or bacteria that can cause cough can also be easily passed on through body fluids so sometimes you can catch it from someone who has it. Other causes of coughs include smoking or inhaling smoke from cigarettes and asthma attacks. Pollution from the environment or dusts can also cause someone to have a cough.

Things to avoid

It is a common adage that *Prevention is always better than cure.* So, as much as possible, try to avoid people who have the virus or, if it you can't help it, maintain minimum contact with them. Always wash your hands after holding or interacting with these people and avoid putting your hands on your mouth. Also avoid sharing utensils with people who have a cough in order to prevent the infection from spreading.

Another thing that you can do in order to make yourself invincible from the virus or bacteria that cause cough is to keep your body healthy. Strengthen your immune system by eating healthy foods, having enough sleep, and exercising regularly.

Remedies

Cough? Mother Nature has an answer to that problem too. There are a lot of herbs and plants that can cure common colds and the best news is that the majority of these plants can be easily found in your home or in your garden. Here are some of the plants that can help you get rid of that terrible cough:

- *Eucalyptus*

  - Eucalyptus has evergreen leaves that are naturally aromatic. Its leaves can be boiled or powdered in order to extract the oil, which can be used for medicine.

    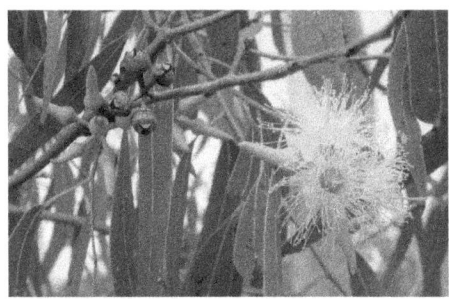

  - The minty taste of its leaves can help relieve throat irritation.

  - Eucalyptus can also be added to rubs for extra cooling effect that can ease difficulty in breathing.

- *Oregano*
  - Our ancestors since time immemorial have been using oregano leaves in order to cure and relieve the symptoms of cough.

    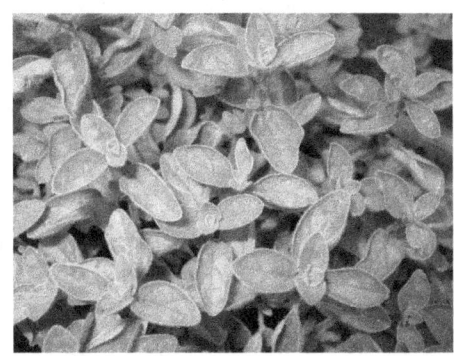

  - You can soak oregano leaves in a cup of boiling water as you would for a bag of tea for a couple of minutes and drink it in order to soften dry cough.

- **Thyme**
  - The Germans have been using thyme as a cure for cough for years.

    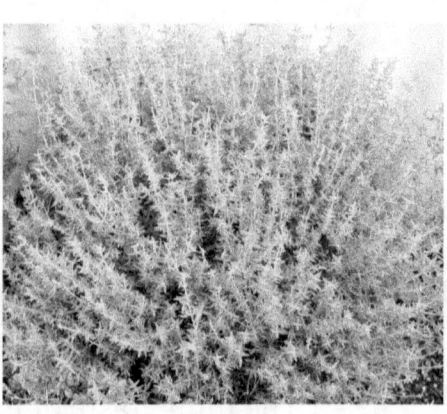

  - Thyme is an herb that contains flavonoids, which relax the muscles in the trachea and can cure inflammation.

  - You can add crushed thyme leaves into water and infuse them for 10 minutes. After it's ready, strain the water and drink.

- **Lemon**
  - Lemon is known for its antiseptic and anti-inflammatory properties.

    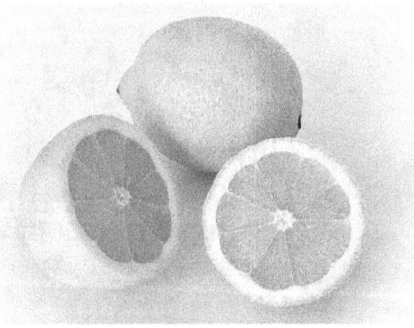

  - It is also a fruit rich in Vitamin C, which helps in fighting colds and cough.

  - To ease throat irritation, you can suck on a quarter of lemon. If it is too sour for you, you can add a little bit of salt to it.

Aside from plants, there are also some practices that can save you from the turmoil of having a cough. For example, you can drink a lot of water to keep your throat from drying up and to make phlegm easier to expel. Rest is very much needed by people who get infected by cough too, so they can recharge and replenish their energy. Sleeping with some extra pillows and elevating your head a little bit can aid in the better passage of air through your lungs to help you breathe smoothly and properly.

Foods to avoid

Stay away from mangos and bananas when you have cough because these fibrous fruits can further irritate your throat. Also avoid milk because it can cause the production of excess mucus, making it stickier and thicker. If you get a cough from asthma, please avoid eggs, nuts, and shellfish like shrimps because these can trigger asthma.

Sore Throat

Just like cold and cough, sore throat is also caused by viral infections. Specifically, it is an infection in the voice box caused by a virus. Its' common symptoms include irritation, pain, or itchiness of the throat, or sometimes a combination of the three. A person who has sore throat may experience difficulty in swallowing, especially crunchy and hard chunks of food. One can also have dry throat, white patches on his or her tonsils, and sometimes, swollen neck glands.

It commonly attacks smokers, kids, and, of course, people with weak immune systems.

Causes

The main cause of sore throat is a virus. However, bacteria and having an unhealthy lifestyle can also be factors. People who live in polluted places or those who consume lots of sweets but don't drink lots of water can be more prone to acquiring sore throat.

Remedies

In curing sore throat, there's no need for expensive gargles and medicines. All you have to do is to mix a pinch of salt with warm water then gargle the mixture for a couple of minutes. You can also relieve the pain in your throat by avoiding cold beverages and drinking warm fluids, like soup, instead, .

First Aid Ointments

There are also natural ointments that can substitute the expensive and synthetic ones in the market. Aside from the fact that these ointments are budget-friendly and can easily be found your surroundings, these are healthy for the body as well. One of the most popular natural ointments is aloe vera, which is a very good cure for burns. The gel that comes from aloe vera has a cooling effect on first-degree burns. Another natural ointment is coconut oil, which can be used as a moisturizer for dry skin and is a cure for boils and wounds. Also, you can use honey for wounds, stings, and minor cuts. Honey is a great antimicrobial and it can help wounds heal faster.

Chapter 2

Natural Remedies For Mental & Neurological Conditions

It is not only minor infections that nature can heal. The environment is so powerful that it extends its healing effects to problems that include our mental and neurological well-being. Here are some tips and cures that will help you battle common emotional and psychological problems without the help of a therapist or a doctor.

Anxiety

Anxiety is an ancient response to harmful stimuli. Our ancestors were constantly surrounded with animals that could hurt or kill them. They had to always be alert in order to escape danger. That response has been passed on to modern men even if our environment is relatively less dangerous than before. Being anxious still benefits us because feeling so heightens our defense mechanisms at times of trouble. But, if we get attacked with anxiety almost regularly, it becomes stressful and unhealthy for us. We become jittery and uneasy while our muscles become tensed.

Although fear and anxiety are both responses related to the "fight or flight" system, fear is different from anxiety in terms of the perception of threat. You feel fear when the threatening stimulus is in front of you but it is anxiety that you feel when you think about a threatening stimulus that can strike you in the future.

How to cure anxiety

The secret to minimize the feeling of being anxious is to always prepare for the future. Sometimes, we become nervous of something because we don't prepare for the possible outcomes that these things can bring. One example is cramming for a major examination. You feel anxious because of the possibility that you might flunk in that examination or it could be failing a job interview or not receiving a promotion. There's a possibility of failure because you didn't study in advance or perform well in the interview. So, for these kinds of circumstances, you can avoid feeling anxious if you plan ahead and prepare for the upcoming stimulus.

If you can't help but feel tensed, you can also have a cup of chamomile tea in order to calm yourself. Chamomile has chemical compounds that can bind together with some receptors in the brain and tell your brain to keep calm and composed. You can also sniff the scent of lavender because it has been proven that doing so can relax tensed muscles and lower your blood pressure to a normal level. Try to eat bananas as well. Bananas have a chemical called tryptophan, which is a precursor to the synthesis of the neurotransmitter called serotonin which can help you feel tranquil and be at peace.

You can also try simple breathing exercises like inhaling and exhaling in order to regulate your breathing. Doing so can also ease muscle tensions and help you feel more relaxed.

Mild Depression

There are just days when we feel so down. This is perfectly normal. We sometimes feel down for no apparent reason because our body cannot sustain being too happy for a long time. Feeling happy all the time is just too energy consuming both for our bodies and our brains. However, prolonged sadness can be very bad for our well-being too. Usually, it takes more than six months for a person to be declared depressed and when that happens, he or she should seek professional help.

How to cure mild depression

Not all forms of depression need to be treated with synthetic drugs. There are natural tips that you can follow to chase the blues away. For example, thinking of happy thoughts. The brain is so powerful that it can dictate your whole body how to behave. You can feel happy by thinking of happy thoughts because doing so can beget more happy thoughts. Avoid people or things that can make you sad and focus on things that make you laugh or smile instead, like a funny book, a comedy show, or a happy classmate. Do not wallow in your sadness and isolate yourself. Doing so will certainly not do you any good and will further drive you to depression.

Another thing that you can do is to perform physical activities as much as possible. Exercising can release certain neurotransmitters in the brain that can help you chase the blues away. Go outside and take a jog with a friend or play some Frisbee. Go walk your dog or take a stroll in the park. You can feel relaxed and one with nature and feel a sense of fulfilment by doing so.

If you feel sad most of the time, make it a habit to let it out. Don't keep all the hurt for yourself. Tell your mom and talk to her about what's bothering you; you can even tell a trusted friend or your pet. Sometimes, people succumb to their depression because they keep all the negativity in and don't have any outlet where they can channel all their sadness.

Insomnia

Insomnia is the inability to sleep soundly and has three different types. A person can have the difficulty to fall fast asleep, have the inability to maintain a sound sleep (waking up unintentionally from time to time), or have the difficulty to go back to sleep after waking up unintentionally.

How to cure insomnia

One of the causes of insomnia is a messed up sleeping pattern so the basic thing that you can do to prevent it is to establish a proper body clock. Make it a habit to sleep and wake up at a specific time. Avoid staying up late or beyond your usual sleeping hours because doing so can confuse your brain and your body when they really want to rest and fall asleep.

Another reason for insomnia is overthinking. Before you go to bed, avoid thinking about mind-boggling mathematical problems, personal problems, or even the mysteries of the earth. Stimulating your brain can increase brain activity, which will lead you to feel energetic. If you have insomnia, try reciting a memorized prayer over and over. Make sure that you don't think too much in order to calm your brain and order your system to fall asleep.

Drinking chamomile tea and taking a hot bath before going to bed can also help you get a good night's sleep. You will feel more relaxed and sleepy afterwards.

Vertigo

People who suffer from vertigo can feel dizzy and, sometimes nauseous. It is as if their environment is constantly spinning or whirling, causing them to lose balance even if they are just standing or sitting still. One of the common causes of vertigo is a damage or infection in the vestibular area of the ear, which give us our sense of balance. When this happens, we lose our composure and feel dizzy or nauseated because of the whirling sensation that we constantly feel. Other causes of vertigo can include eye problems, brain tumor, head injuries and heart problems, dehydration, and anemia.

How to cure vertigo

First and foremost, you need to have enough sleep because skipping on much needed sleep can lead to the symptoms of vertigo just like dizziness. Having enough sleep can also keep you from being anaemic.

If you ever suddenly feel dizzy, make sure that you sit or lie down at once to avoid falling down and hitting your head on the floor. After doing such, try to rest your head between your legs in order to facilitate faster blood flow through the brain.

Since vertigo is also caused by dehydration, you must make sure that you constantly keep your body hydrated by drinking lots of fluids. Juices, soups, and energy drinks can be helpful as well.

Another thing that you can do to cure your vertigo is to stand up or move gently. Abrupt body movements can only exacerbate the feeling of being dizzy and being sick. You can also try inhaling some minty rubs or liniments that have the aroma of menthol. This can help you feel less sick and less dizzy.

Chapter 3

Natural Remedies For Gastrointestinal Conditions

We all love to eat and eating is one of the simple joys in which almost all human beings indulge. We love to eat comfort food whenever we feel sad, lonely, or broken hearted. Food is even a requisite in any social gathering or activity. Eating is a major part of our day-to-day lives since we acquire the necessary nutrients and minerals that our body needs through the consumption of food. However, food consumption becomes less enjoyable when problems that involve our digestive system hit us. We don't get to appreciate our delicious food well whenever we have these kinds of problems.

We don't have to worry though because surprisingly, there are also natural remedies and cures for gastrointestinal problems. The healing effects of nature do not only cover problems that involve the brain and mild infections caused by bacteria and viruses but it also have available solution for our tummy problems.

Diarrhea

Diarrhoea happens when the large intestines fail to extract fluids or water, which leads to a watery stool. When someone has diarrhoea, he or she frequently goes to the bathroom and his or her faeces are accompanied by lots of water. Bacteria, viruses, or food poisoning can cause it.

Remedies

When you suffer from diarrhoea, make sure that you frequently rehydrate by drinking lots of water to prevent the loss of a lot of electrolytes. You can also eat yogurt in order to increase the number of healthy bacteria that will facilitate in good digestion. Also munch on bananas, toast, and rice in order to soothe your upset stomach. Bananas contain a soluble fibre that can slow down the passage of stool. This fibre can also be found in carrots so you can also munch on those if you prefer.

Constipation

Constipation is characterized by difficult and less frequent bowel movements. Someone who is suffering this can experience pain and difficulty in removing bowels because of hardened stool, which was caused by too much absorption of water by the colon.

The common causes of constipation include low fibre content in one's diet, inactivity, not drinking enough water, and impeding bowel movement.

Remedies

The main solution to constipation is to eat lots of fibrous fruits and green leafy vegetables like papaya, mangoes, and moringa olifera. Fibre is the natural sweeper in our colon and it helps in the faster digestion of our food. Yogurt is also a very good food to eat whenever you have constipation because it promotes the growth of good bacteria in the colon, which are also helpful in digestion. Aside from water, you can also opt for prune juice, which is rich in fibre and contains sorbitol, which softens stool. Drinking lemon juice can also be helpful since its citric acid component stimulates the digestive system.

Bloating & Gas

It is natural for us to pass gas through flatulence and burping. They our body's ways of getting rid of swallowed air and telling us that the food we've consumed have already been broken down. But, there are times when we can't belch or pass gas that's why we become bloated.

Remedies

Eating too many fatty foods and eating too fast can also cause bloating. To prevent bloating, try to eat and chew your food slowly. This allows your tummy to get ready to process that food and doing so will also enable you to enjoy your food better. You should also try to avoid carbonated drinks like sodas because these can increase the amount of air in your stomach and cause bloating.

Nausea

We feel sick or feel like we are about to vomit because of a lot of reasons. Usually, vomiting is a sign that you've been hit by another disease just like the flu or a fever. Vomiting is also our body's way of getting rid of toxic and stale food that we have unconsciously and accidentally ate.

Remedies

Vomiting can also translate to losing water and electrolytes. So, it is only imperative that you replenish lost bodily fluids by drinking lots of water. Another remedy for nausea is eating soda crackers in order to absorb the excess acids in your stomach. Applying pressure on your palm also helps in stopping the feeling of being sick.

Chapter 4

Natural Remedies Skin & External Conditions

Diseases don't only attack us from the inside, but mess up with our skin too. Here are some of the natural ways in which you can prevent common skin problems and conditions.

Sunburn

When we stay too long under the heat of the sun, we become overexposed to its harmful rays, causing our skin to get a little inflamed and burnt.

Remedies

To soothe your inflamed skin, you can try applying aloe vera gel, which is very good in soothing burns, cucumber slices or a cold compress on the burnt areas. These will ease the painful sensation and reduce inflammation. You can also apply oatmeal soaked on cold water or a mixture of cornstarch and water on the burnt area in order to relieve yourself from the painful and stinging sensation.

Avoid using soap for a few days too because soap can further dry up your skin and exacerbate the redness and pain.

Toenail Fungus

This condition is caused by fungus and it causes the nail to become discoloured, broken, or damaged. This is also hard to cure since toenails grow slowly which consequently lead to the bacteria spreading easily.

Remedies

To get rid of this nasty infection, you can soak your feet in apple cider vinegar or apply tea tree oil in the affected are. Apple cider vinegar can avoid the spread of the fungus because of its acidic property while tea tree oil has antiseptic and anti-fungal properties.

Puffy Eyes

Puffy eyes can be caused by the irritation and itchiness in the skin around the eye. A few culprits behind this are allergies, the lack of sleep, or even stress.

Remedies

Drinking lots of water can get rid of puffy eyes by flushing out the excess water that causes some body parts to swell. Tea bags and slices of cucumber are helpful as well, as they soothe swelling and have anti-inflammatory properties and can also help relax the eye muscles.

Rash

Rashes can sometimes occur whenever allergens or bacteria that cause these diseases irritate our skin. The symptoms of rash that you should watch out for are itchy, chapped, and scaly skin.

Remedies

Vitamin C is very important in treating rashes since it brings back the firmness and the moisture of the skin. So, be sure to eat fruits like lemon and oranges because these are known fruits that are abundant in Vitamin C. You can also wash the infected area with chamomile tea, oatmeal, and aloe vera in order to reduce itchiness and in order to moisturize torn skin.

Eczema

Eczema is a painful skin condition that's characterized by rough and inflamed patches on the skin, which are often accompanied by blisters.

Remedies

The oil extracted from sweet almonds can be used as cure for rashes because it contains Vitamin C. Natural skin moisturizers can also be found in coconut oil and aloe vera, which can ease the discomfort of having dry and scaly skin caused by eczema.

Psoriasis

Psoriasis is a chronic skin problem that is characterized by thick, white or red patches on the skin. This is caused by the abnormally fast growth of the skin cells.

Remedies

There are studies that support that claim that avoiding fatty foods, as well as red meat can help cure eczema. Olive oil, coconut oil, aloe vera, and apple cider vinegar can help with the itchiness, the inflammation, and the dryness of the skin because of their anti-inflammatory, anti-fungal, and antiseptic properties.

Chapter 5

Natural Remedies For Daily Ailments

There are also diseases that may not cause us to be bed-ridden but still cause a great deal of inconvenience like heartburn, joint pain, headache, menstrual cramps, yeast infections, and muscle pains. Here are some ways on how you can remedy these problems.

Heartburn

Heartburn is a burning feeling in the chest area caused by too much acidity in your stomach and indigestion. Mixing a spoonful of baking soda in water in order to neutralize the acidic state of your stomach can easily cure this. You can also eat some bananas or apples because they have natural antacids that remedy hyperacidity. Surprisingly, chewing gum is also considered a cure for heartburn because doing so can stimulate the salivary glands to produce more saliva in order to get rid of the excess acid in your stomach.

Joint Pain

Joint pains are also known as soreness in the joints. It is common in aged individuals and people who either had too much exercise or those who don't exercise at all. You can cure the inflammation of your joints by using ginger tea. You can also massage virgin olive oil on your sore muscles in order to relax them and ease the pain. It is also important that you munch on spinach, nuts, and legumes because these foods are rich in magnesium that can help prevent sore muscles and joints. Exercising regularly also helps too because doing so can loosen the joints and enable you to move easier.

Headaches

There are numerous ways on how you can relieve yourself from headache. You can massage your temples in order to release certain neurotransmitters that act as natural painkillers. Sometimes, headaches are caused by stress. In order to cure it, you can try getting out to inhale some fresh air and relax yourself. You can also look or focus on something green like a leaf or a plant since doing so can give you the feeling of being relaxed.

Menstrual Cramps

Menstrual cramps are something that most women can relate to. It is caused by contractions in the uterus and this usually occurs during the onset of menstruation. Its symptoms include pain or pressure in the abdomen.

You can ease the pain by taking a warm bath and doing some exercise like yoga.

Yeast Infection

One the most common vaginal infection that women acquire is the yeast infection. It is caused by the overgrowth of fungus in the vagina. Luckily, this is highly curable. You can eat yogurt in order to help the good bacteria in the vagina grow in number and fight the fungus. You can also rely on garlic for its anti-fungal properties and place a clove of garlic on your lady part while sleeping.

Muscle Pain

Watermelon juice has been proven to treat muscle pains because it contains an amino acid called l-citrulline that fights muscle pain. You can also opt for a warm bath or a nice massage in order to relax the muscles. You can drink a mixture of some apple cider vinegar and water too for muscle relaxation.

Chapter 6

Natural Health & Skin Care Recipes For Children Under 12

Children have relatively a weaker immune system than adults. They need special care and attention so that they will not easily acquire illnesses and diseases. Their skin is highly sensitive too and prone to skin infections and complications.

Here are some simple tips to protect your child from the threat of infection and diseases.

1. ### *Make sure that your child is eating a balanced diet.*

Diet is everything. Eating the right kinds of food can help your child reach his or her full potentials and can protect him or her from being hit with terrible illnesses. Make sure that your kid is eating healthily and keeping a supply of fruits and vegetables. He or she needs to have the three major food groups in every meal too to acquire the essential nutrients and minerals that are needed by the body. Discourage your child from eating junk and fatty foods.

1. ### *Let your child exercise regularly.*

Make sure that your child doesn't get too caught up with video games and the Internet and still have them go out and play outside. Go out with your children for a run or a stroll in the park as a boding session.

2. ***Teach your child to observe proper hygiene.***

Let your child understand that the key to avoiding diseases is by observing cleanliness in his or her body and in the surroundings. Teach your children the importance of hand washing before and after every meal. Make sure that they take a bath every day and that they change into dry and clean clothes after playing outside to prevent rashes or the spread of bacteria.

Natural Skin Care Recipes

Before applying any natural skin care remedy, you have to research and read up on your ingredients or the herbs that you are going to use. Make sure that you have substantial information about the plants just to be safe.

You can make natural moisturizers by mixing an emulsifier with water and a kind of oil of your choice. Just make sure that your child is not allergic to the oil that you're going to use.

You can also extract coconut oil from coconut juice or water by heating the juice for more or less 1 hour, until the juice becomes crystal clear. Coconut oil is gentle for the skin and is great in treating dryness.

Conclusion

It is very comforting to know that we have an environment that could provide us with natural cures that don't introduce harmful toxins to our bodies. It is also great to know that some of the common diseases that we suffer from can be treated without having to take synthetic medicines.

Hopefully, this ebook inspired you to try out some of the natural cures that can serve as alternative to synthetic drugs and encouraged you to make your own homemade first aid.

From The Author

Thank you for taking the time to read this book. As an author, I understand the importance of creating books which my readers will find both enjoyable and informative. If you have the time and feel generous, please don't hesitate to leave an honest review of this book.........*Dr Alex Nelson·*

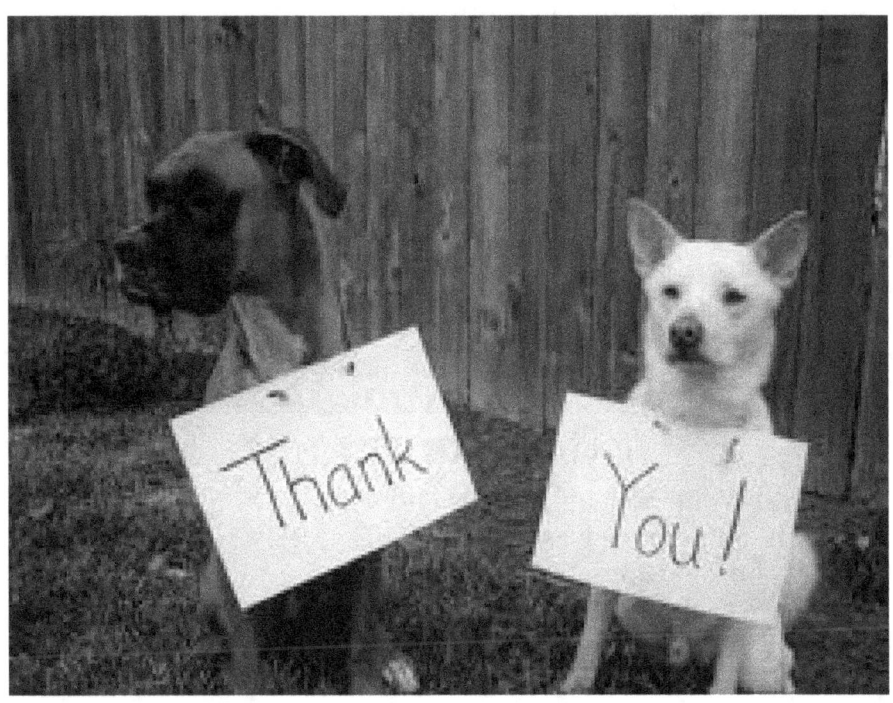

Other Books By Dr Alex Nelson

Cure Adrenal Fatigue Now!

Adrenal Fatigue doesn't have to control your life. There are solutions to help you diagnose and overcome this modern day symptom of stress. Within the pages of this easy-to-read guide, Dr. Alex Nelson, has outlined all the information you need to know in order to combat the dreaded listlessness and show you the steps necessary to recharge your energy levels and leave you feeling invigorated and ready for any of life's challenges. Discover the natural remedies that can and will change your life.

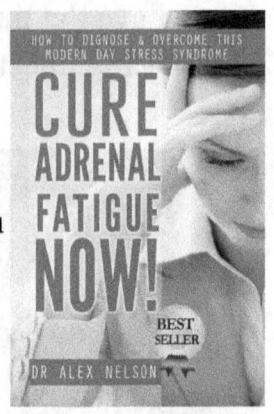

Natural Antibiotics And Antivirals For Beginners

The world is rife with antibiotics and antivirals. What once was non existent, now, has become commonplace. Having an abundance to these substances doesn't equate to overall general health or cures for minor ailments. Inside the pages of this book, you will find detailed descriptions, weighing the pros and cons of synthetic products versus natural products. Discover the secrets behind creating your own natural antibiotics inexpensively while keeping your health and well-being in

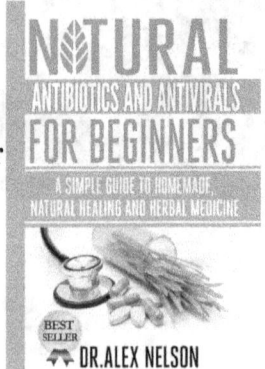

mind. Not only will you find recipes for antibiotics, but you will also find tips and tricks for natural oils, antivirals, natural skin remedies and more.

www.ingramcontent.com/pod-product-compliance
Lightning Source LLC
Chambersburg PA
CBHW070523290526
45790CB00003B/1276